Organic Perfume:

55 Ultimate Recipes For Beginners - Learn How To Make Aromatic, Non-Toxic Organic Fragrances At Home!

Copyright 2016 - All rights reserved.

This document is geared towards providing exact and reliable information in regards to the topic and issue covered. The publication is sold with the idea that the publisher is not required to render legal, financial, medical or any professional services. If advice is necessary, legal or professional, a practiced individual in the profession should be ordered.

In no way is it legal to reproduce, duplicate, or transmit any part of this document in either electronic means or in printed format. Recording of this publication is strictly prohibited and any storage of this document is not allowed unless with written permission from the publisher. All rights reserved.

The information provided herein is stated to be truthful and consistent, in that any liability, in terms of inattention or otherwise, by any usage or abuse of any policies, processes, or directions contained within is the solitary and utter responsibility of the recipient reader. Under no circumstances will any legal responsibility or blame be held against the publisher for any reparation, damages, or monetary loss due to the information herein, either directly or indirectly.

The information herein is offered for informational purposes solely, and is universal as so. The presentation of the information is without contract or any type of guarantee assurance.

The trademarks that are used are without any consent, and the publication of the trademark is without permission or backing by the trademark owner. All trademarks and brands within the book are for clarifying purposes only and are owned by the owners themselves, not affiliated with this document.

Table Of Contents

Organic Perfume:

Introduction

Chapter 1 – Introduction to Making Organic Perfumes

Chapter 2 – Essential Oils

Chapter 3 – What You Need

Chapter 4 – Blending Fragrances

Chapter 5 – Organic Perfume Recipes

Chapter 6 – Solid Perfume

Chapter 7 – Aromatherapy

Conclusion

Handwritten notes:
3 Categories
Cleaning product fragrance
home fragrance
personal fragrance

Introduction

Organic perfumes are made of all natural botanical oils, such as essential oils and absolutes. More and more people are moving toward do-it-yourself organic perfumes instead of expensive store bought perfumes. Let's talk about why people are opting for organic perfume instead of commercial perfumes.

Chemicals

With organic perfume, you don't have to worry about having potentially harmful, man-made chemicals in your perfume. The fragrances you wear will be natural, and some will have potential health benefits, too. All the scents and fragrances in your perfume will be natural, not synthetic.

For example, suppose a perfume you buy at the store says it contains jasmine. It might contain a tiny amount of real jasmine, but most of the jasmine scent comes from synthetic aromas produced in a laboratory.

Health

The synthetic ingredients often lead to allergic reactions and severe headaches, too. To make matters worse, some of the synthetic ingredients also act as hormone disruptors. Many fragrances also contain ingredients aren't listed on the bottle.

Some independent researchers have tested this unlisted ingredients, and discovered that over time some ingredients can accumulate in human tissue, which is definitely not a good thing. Many of these ingredients have never been tested for adverse effects, and those that have been tested are usually tested on animals.

Animals

That leads to concerns about animal testing and exploitation. Did you know that even animal-based musk scents can be reproduced using essential oils? And when using essential oils, there is no need to test them on animals, so your scents will be 100% animal-friendly, in every sense of the word.

Environment

Your perfume will also be environmentally friendly, and do far less damage to the environment than commercial fragrances. Most commercial perfumes contain petrochemicals that are by-products of processing crude oil. Again, the ingredients in organic perfumes are natural, without any dangerous chemical by-products produced during their processing.

Cost

Another plus is that most organic perfumes are less expensive than their store-bought. The supplies needed are easy to find locally or online, and aren't expensive. They are very easy to make, too.

Personalization

Finally, the perfume will be one of a kind, and reflect you own personal tastes and preferences. Imagine having your very own fragrance! Not only that, but you can customize fragrances for loved ones as gifts they won't soon forget.

Aromatherapy

One last benefit of organic perfumes made with essential oils is aromatherapy: essential oils can have positive effects on your emotions. By combining essential oils not just for fragrance but for their aromatherapy effects, you can have a perfume that lifts your mood or relaxes you.

So, are you ready to jump into the world of organic perfumes? Let's start with an overview of how it's done.

Chapter 1 – Introduction to Making Organic Perfumes

This is a very abstract, simple introduction on how to make organic perfume using essential oils. We will go into more detail about ingredients, equipment, and steps later on.

The goal of this chapter is simply to provide you an overview, a rough structure of understanding to build upon. We will start with the four basic ingredients and what they do, then talk about the basic process.

Ingredients

There are four basic ingredients to the typical organic perfume:

1. **Carrier oil** (sweet almond, grape seed, jojoba, fractionated coconut oil)
2. **Essential oils** (source of the scent)
3. **Pure gain alcohol** (80- to 100-proof vodka recommended)
4. **Distilled water** or bottled spring water

The **carrier oil** serves to dilute the essential oils, and oil is necessary because oil and water don't mix very well. If not diluted, the essential oils will most likely irritate your skin. In short, it safely "carries" the scent of the essential oils.

The scent is provided through a blend of two or more **essential oils**. Natural essential oils can be found health food stores, as well as numerous places online.

The purpose of the **pure grain alcohol** is to help the oils merge together to form a blend. Alcohol is used for this because it evaporates quickly. You'll notice that vodka is recommended -- many perfumers use high quality vodka (and the higher the proof, the less natural vodka scent remains).

The **bottled water** is used to dilute the final fragrance to an acceptable strength of scent.

Basic Process

The basic procedure for creating an organic perfume from essential oils is as follows:

- Combine the essential oils with the carrier oil.
- Mix these with pure grain alcohol.
- Let the mixture cure for anywhere from 48 hours to 1 month. The longer the mixture stands, the stronger the resulting fragrance will be – this is the curing step.
- After the mixture has been left standing, add about two tablespoons of the distilled water/spring water to dilute the mixture. You can add more water as needed to achieve the level of dilution you want.

- Now your perfume is ready to use!

Optional Ingredients

You can also add a tablespoon of glycerin to you mix so that the fragrance will last longer. Glycerin is a thick, colorless, neutral liquid that helps the other perfume ingredients to dissolver faster and better, and make the scent last longer. You can usually find glycerin anyplace that sells soapmaking supplies, including online sellers.

Chapter 2 – Essential Oils

Essential oils are the source of scent in your organic perfume. This chapter will cover the basics of what you need to get a running start with using essential oils. We'll start with talking about what essential oils are, and how they can differ from other oils like fragrance oils or absolutes. We'll also discuss carrier oils and fixatives, ending with a discussion on how to safely use essential oils.

What Are Essential Oils?

Essential oils are all-natural plant extracts. They come from the flowers, stems, roots, fruit, or bark of plants, and are extracted by methods such as pressing or steam distillation, which don't require any dangerous chemicals. Many essential oils have desirable aromas, and most have additional therapeutic benefits we'll discuss in a later chapter on aromatherapy.

What about Fragrance or Perfume Oils?

You will also see potpourri oils, perfume oils, and fragrance oils. Their scents are weaker, and some may be artificially produced. If the bottle is labeled fragrance oils or synthetic oils, or includes additional ingredients, it is not an essential oil and is not recommended for use in your organic perfume. Stick to 100% pure essential oils.

What about Absolutes or CO2s?

Strictly speaking, absolutes are essential oils. The difference is how they are extracted from the plant: absolutes are extracted using solvents and may contain traces of that solvent.

This causes issues if you are aiming for an organic perfume free of artificial ingredients and extra chemicals. Also be aware that they will be much more concentrated than essential oils.

CO2s are extracted from the plants using pressurized CO_2, which turns into a liquid and acts as a solvent to extract the oils. Unlike absolutes, the CO_2 solvent evaporates completely, leaving behind no trace of solvent. CO2s are usually much thicker than essential oils, and don't mix well for purposes of making perfumes.

What are Carrier Oils?

As already mentioned, carrier oils are used to dilute the essential oils ... but they also serve a secondary, and even more important purpose: they "carry" the oils and their scent when you spray the perfume on. Typical carrier oils used in organic perfume are sweet almond, grape seed, jojoba, and fractionated coconut oil.

The reason essential oils need to be diluted is because they are very strong. For 20% dilution, you would use one part essential oil to four parts carrier oil. For 10% dilution, try one part essential oil to nine parts carrier oil.

For example, if you are using a total of five drops of essential oils, then you would need 20 drops of carrier oil to achieve 20% dilution. You can always add more carrier oil to reduce the strength of the essential oils.

What Essential Oils are Recommended for Beginners?

One of the most expensive essential oils should come as no surprise: rose oil. Fifteen milliliters of 100% pure rose essential oil requires 65 pounds of rose petals, and the cost would be over $500. However, most essential oils are not that expensive!

For beginners, or those with a limited budget, these are your best bets to start out with: cedarwood, chamomile, geranium, ginger, grapefruit, lavender, lemon, mint, neroli, sweet orange, and ylang ylang.

What are Fixatives?

Fixatives are heavier oils that help your fragrance to last longer. The most commonly used fixative oils are ylang ylang, sandalwood, and myrrh. They not only add a pleasant accent to your fragrance, but make it last longer. However, there is a limit to how much staying power they can add to a fragrance.

Proper Care of Essential Oils

Essential oils should always be stored in dark glass containers away from direct sunlight. Because essential oils can degrade rubber, don't store your essential oils with a rubber stopper or dropper.

Health and Safety

Even though essential oils are all natural, that doesn't mean you won't ever have a reaction to them. If you are allergic to a certain plant in daily life, you'll probably be allergic to it as an essential oils. If you aren't sure whether or not you'll be allergic to one, do a small patch test on your skin. Next, pregnant women should avoid using essential oils.

Here are essential oils that have a reputation for causing skin irritation: Bay Laurel, Cassia, Cinnamon, Clove, Fennel, Fir Needle, Sage, Spruce, and Thyme. These essential oils can cause skin sensitization: Cassia, Cinnamon, Clove, Fennel, Lemongrass, Melissa, Oakmoss, Pine.

These are some of the essential oils that can react with sunlight: Bergamot, Grapefruit, Lemon, Lime. If you dilute your essential oils properly by mixing them with a carrier oil, this should not be a problem.

Chapter 3 – What You Need

This chapter covers more detail on what you need to setup your own organic perfume laboratory. We'll start with basic equipment, followed by ingredients. We'll also review the purpose of the ingredients.

Equipment

Let's get started with a discussion on the equipment you need. Latex gloves are useful for keeping essential oils off your hands, where they can last much, much longer that you would expect – especially in their pure, undiluted form. This is also good if you have sensitive skin or are prone to skin allergies.

To test your fragrances before you mix an entire batch, it's a good idea to have fragrance blotters, cotton balls, or coffee filters on hand. These quickly absorb the oil and allow you to smell it. You can try out your blends this way, to make sure they smell like you are expecting.

When blending the oils, you should add them a drop at a time. Most essential oils also come with reducer caps, which prevents you from pouring out too much at a time. Glass droppers or pipettes work very well for controlling how many drops of an oil you are adding to a blend, and much better than the reducer caps.

For the highest level of accuracy, droppers and pipettes are recommended. Again, glass should be used instead of plastic because essential oils can degrade plastic and rubber.

You'll need a small glass container for blending the oils, and a storage container to allow the oils to cure in. Both should be glass, and the storage container should be amber or dark blue to prevent exposure to light, which can weaken the oils.

For applying your perfume, you should have a glass spray bottle, spritzer bottle, vintage perfume bottle, or a glass roll-on container. You can also find vintage style perfume bottles online. All of these can easily be found online.

You also should have a funnel for pouring the fragrance into the spray bottle. Many perfumers also use a coffee filter (or similar filter) with the funnel to strain the fragrance.

Labels are a must, but easily overlooked. Make sure that your bottles of perfume, both when curing and in their final form, are clearly labeled. Inexpensive labels are not difficult to find, or you can opt for a solution such as a label-maker.

On a practical note, you should also have a notebook to keep track of all your essential oils recipes, especially those that you develop yourself. Trust us – you'll kick yourself if you come up with a wonderful fragrance but can't remember the ingredients!

Ingredients

You need a good selection of essential oils, of course. As already discussed, 100% pure essential oils are recommended if you want a truly natural, organic perfume. They are stronger than fragrance oils, and do not contain leftover chemicals from distillation like absolutes. They are less viscous than CO2s, making them easier to work with.

You also need a good supply of carrier oils, as well as bottled spring or distilled water. Good carrier oils include jojoba and fractionated coconut oil. Remember that the carrier oils prevent skin irritation and help carry your fragrance. The water is used to dilute the final fragrance as needed.

High-proof vodka is needed to enable the oils to blend. Remember that the higher-proof vodkas will not have a strong vodka scent, and are more desirable when making your perfumes. All of these ingredients should be easy enough to find at your local grocery store or drug store.

Chapter 4 – Blending Fragrances

In this chapter, we are going to look at some of the different approaches perfumers take in combining scents to create awesome fragrances. We'll start with the concept of perfume notes, then discuss aroma categories. Next we'll look at season scents followed by chypres. We'll end with a few notes on background scents.

Perfume Notes

There is a science behind developing fragrances, and one of the foundational concepts is perfume notes. Perfume notes represent the phases that a fragrance goes through as it begins to evaporate from your skin. Notes exist because oils evaporate at different speeds. There are three notes in perfumes: a top note, a middle note, and a base note.

Base notes last about 4 to 5 hours, top notes last about 10 to 15 minutes, and middle notes last somewhere in between. Top notes are what you smell first from a fragrance, and are usually the strongest. They are used to "top off" the fragrance blend.

Middle notes are also referred to as the heart note because they form the heart of the fragrance. They are usually soothing (as opposed to pungent), and typically chosen from among floral scents. The base note accentuates the middle note. Their scent is heavier, musky, and thicker.

As a beginner, you should stick with just three oils: one for the base note, one for the middle note, and one for the top note. The table below summarizes which essential oils are associated with which fragrance notes. Some essential oils may be associated with more than one fragrance note.

Base	Middle	Top
Ambrette seed	Bay	Anise
Angelica	Black pepper	Basil
Balsam	Bois-de-rose	Bay laurel
Benzoin	Cajeput	Bergamot
Cassia	Carrot seed	Bergamot mint
Cedarwood	Cardamom	Citronella
Clove	Chamomile	Coriander
Cypress	Cinnamon	Eucalyptus
Frankincense	Clary sage	Galbanum
Ginger	Cypress	Grapefruit
Helichrysum	Dill	Lavender
Jasmine	Elemi	Lavendin
Myrrh	Fennel	Lemon
Oakmoss	Fir needle	Lemongrass
Olibanum	Geranium	Lime
Patchouli	Hyssop	Mandarin
Sandalwood	Juniper berry	Neroli
Vanilla	Linden blossom	Orange
Vetiver	Marjoram	Peppermint
	Melissa	Rosemary

	Myrtle	Spearmint
	Neroli	Sweet orange
	Nutmeg	Tangerine
	Palmarosa	Thyme
	Parsley	
	Rose	
	Rose Geranium	
	Rosemary	
	Rosewood	
	Scotch pine	
	Sweet orange	
	Spruce	
	Tea Tree	
	Tobacco	
	Violet leaf	
	Yarrow	
	Ylang Ylang	

When you combine the oils to make a fragrance blend, start with adding the base notes, followed by the middle and top notes. There are several different opinions as to how to properly ratio base-middle-top notes, but here are three commonly used methods:

- 1 drop base, 2 drops middle, 3 drops top
- 50% base, 20% middle, 30% top
- 65% base, 20% middle, and 15% top

There is another approach to combining essential oils for fragrances. Essential oils scents can also be classified as personifiers, enhancers, equalizers, and modifies. Personifiers make up to 5% of the blend have strong, sharp aromas like clary sage or clove.

Enhances make up 505 to 80% of the fragrance and are the dominant scents, such as Melissa. Equalizers are between 10% and 51% of the fragrance blend and are used to balance the scent out. They don't last as long as enhancers or personifiers.

A good example of an equalizer would be oregano or melaleuca alternifolia. Finally, the modifers constitute between 5% and 8% of the fragrance blend and are used to harmonize the scent. Grapefruit is a commonly used modifier.

Aroma Categories

There are different ways of categorizing aromas related to essential oils. One classification is given below, where oils in the same category are known to blend well together. Note that some scents can belong to more than one category.

Category	Typical essential oils
Citrus	Lemon, lime, sweet orange, tangerine, grapefruit, and bergamot
Earthy	Sandalwood, patchouli, valerian, vetiver, and oakmoss

Floral	Jasmine, lavender, rose, chamomile, geranium, neroli, and ylang ylang
Herbaceous	Basil, hyssop, clary sage, melissa, chamomile, rosemary, marjoram, and lavender
Camphorous	Eucalyptus, cajuput, rosemary, and tea tree
Resinous	Elemi, frankincense, myrrh
Minty	Spearmint, peppermint, and wintergreen
Spicy	Black pepper, coriander, cumin, ginger, cinnamon, nutmeg, clove, and cardamom
Woodsy	Pine, sandalwood, cedar, cypress, juniper berry

Here are some other tips on blending based on these categories:

- Camphorous + Woodsy
- Earthy + Woodsy
- Earthy + Minty
- Spicy + Floral
- Spicy + Woodsy
- Spicy + Citrus
- Floral + Woodsy
- Floral + spicy
- Floral + citrus
- Herbaceous + Woodsy
- Herbaceous + Minty
- Minty + Woodsy
- Minty + Earthy
- Minty + Herbaceous
- Minty + Citrus

- Citrus + Floral
- Citrus + Minty
- Citrus + Spicy
- Citrus + Woodsy

Seasonal

Essential oils can also be classified by season.

Season	Essential Oils
Spring	bergamot, cardamom, clary sage, dill, eucalyptus, chamomile (german or roman), grapefruit, jasmine, lavender, lemongrass, lime, marjoram, Melissa, orange, rose, rosewood, tea tree, ylang ylang
Summer	bergamot, clary sage, fennel, geranium, ginger, grapefruit, jasmine, lavender, lemon, lime, orange, marjoram, neroli, patchouli, chamomile (roman), sandalwood, spearmint, cedarwood, ylang ylang
Fall	cardamom, bay, cassia, cedarwood, cinnamon, clove bud, coriander, dill, fennel, frankincense, scotch pine, sweet orange, ginger, myrrh, nutmeg, oakmoss, peppermint, patchouli, rosewood, sage, vanilla, vetiver
Winter	bay, cardamom, cassia, cedarwood, peppermint, cinnamon, clove, sage, dill, fir needle, ginger, juniper, myrhh, nutmeg, oakmos, peppermint, scotch pine, spruce, sweet orange, vanilla, vetiver

Chypres

Another classification is by chypres, which is one of the oldest methods of developing fragrances. Classic chypre perfumes combine four key scents: bergamot, oakmoss, patchouli, and labdanum.

Modern variations use bergamot for the top note with oakmoss and patchouli for the bottom note, and then your choice of scents for the middle notes, based on these types of chypres.

Type of Chypres	Essential Oils Used
Animalic	Black currant, valerian, angelica
Coniferous	Cedar leaf, pine needle, scotch pine, cypress
Floral	Jasmine, rose, neroli, lavender, ylang ylang, orange blossom
Fresh	Lemon, lime, tangerine, sweet orange, grapefruit, petitgrain, melissa, lemon verbena
Green/Herbal	Basil, geranium, tarragon, helichrysum, chamomile, hyssop, bay laurel, clary sage
Leather	Angelica, birch tara, cade, choya loban
Woody	Atlas cedarwood, agarwood, sandalwood, corianger, vetiver, carrot seed, rosewood, araucaria

Background Scents

There is one more additional approach to combining scents. First, pick a primary scent and then add one or two background scents. Good background scents include clary sage, cedar, ylang ylang, orange, or ginger.

Developing Your Own Scents

This chapter contains the detailed procedure for how to properly create your own perfume. It also includes some hints and tips to help you along. It ends with some information on how to properly clean the glassware you use, which can be tricky when working with essential oils.

Some Things to Keep in Mind

First, be aware that what might initially smell fantastic can change over time. Give your mixture time to set before you commit to making an entire bottle of it to be sure that you approve of the different aromas it provides over time as the individual essential oils begin to evaporate.

Your organic perfumes will likely not last as long as store-bought perfumes because they don't contain the artificial chemicals that can give them additional staying power. The use of fixatives, as we've have already mentioned, can extend the staying power of your fragrance, but not indefinitely.

Detailed Procedure

Here is a the detailed procedure. You need to use about 30% essential oil and 70% alcohol (vodka). After curing, you need about 5% bottled water or spring water.

- Measure 1 tablespoon of carrier oil into a glass container.

- Add your essential oils to the carrier oil one drop at a time, beginning with the base notes, followed by middle notes, and then the top notes.

- Stir or shake only after you have added all your essential oils.

- Add the alcohol (as mentioned, 80- to 100-proof Vodka is recommended) and thin blend the mixture by stirring or shaking.

- Put the lid on the glass bottle.

- Allow it to cure for anywhere from 2 to 30 days. Don't keep opening the bottle to smell the mixture, or you will cause it to lose its strength.

- Once the curing is complete, add a single tablespoon of bottled water or spring water to dilute the fragrance. Tap water is not

- Once the fragrance has cured, add 1 tablespoon of distilled water or bottled spring water to dilute the fragrance. Tap water is not acceptable. If the scent is still too strong, add a bit more water to the mixture.

- Close the lid and shake to mix thoroughly.

- Pour the mixture into a glass perfume or spritzer bottle. Its best to pour the mixture through a coffee filter and into a funnel to prevent messy spills.

- Label the bottle, and its ready to use!

What if we add too much of something? If you add a drop too much of a scent, many perfumers feel that adding a few drops of orange oil will cancel it out its effects.

You can clean the glass container by washing it in extremely hot water and then place it in a baking pan to dry it in the oven at 230°F.

Chapter 5 – Organic Perfume Recipes

This chapter contains a variety of recipes to get your started on creating your own perfume, and to inspire you own creations!

Two-Scent

This recipe is based on using two simple scents: clove and lavender, rose and cypress, or ylang ylang and sweet orange.

- **Spicy Scent**

    Here's a recipe with a spicy hint to it, with a base of grapefruit.

    - Base note: 10 drops grapefruit   *not commercial perfume*
    - Middle note: 14 drops ginger
    - Top note: 10 drops vetiver

- **Exotically Simple Scent**   *Personal Fragrance*

    Here's an exotic scent with just three essential oils that's guaranteed to please.

    - Base note: 4 drops patchouli
    - Middle note: 8 drops rose

(1)
- Top note: 12 drops lavender

Rose Scent

This recipe is for a pleasant floral scent with a strong scent of rose.

- Base note 25 drops rose
- Middle note: 10 drops lime
- Top note: 10 drops vetiver

✓★
Sweet and Spicy Scent Home Scent | Personal Fragrance

Are you in the mood for something sweet and spicy? Try this recipe, that includes a woody hint of scent.

- (3) Base note: 20 drops sweet orange
- (2) Middle note: 15 drops ylang ylang
- (1) Top note: 10 drops cedarwood

Lavender Dreams Home Scent

This is a wonderful scent to use at night.

- Base note: 4 drops rosemary
- Middle note: 8 drops lemon

- Top note: 12 drops lavender

Hyper dense Scentual Blends

✻ Floral Garden Scent

If you love flowers, you'll love this wonderful blend of botanical essential oils.

- Base note: 10 drops cedarwood
- Base note: 10 drops patchouli
- Middle note: 5 drops ylang ylang
- Top note: 5 drops lavender
- Top note: 20 drops sweet orange
- Top note: 5 drops bergamot

website could have a "winter theme" subtle

What would a more masculine floral be like?

darker flowers bloom in the fall or winter — denser florals

✓ ✻ Gypsies — Personal Fragrances

Here's a mysterious, spicy scent.

- ⓘ Base note: 2 drops vanilla
- ⓘ Base note: 2 drops clove
- ⓘ Middle note: 8 drops nutmeg
- ⓘ Top note: 12 drops lavender

something needed to make it a little more mysterious

I might give this a strong amber base & use the florals? Spice as modifiers ← lavender

✓ ✻ Sandalwood Memories — Personal Fragrances

Could you put a vanilla bean in a perfume?

Here's a fascinating sandalwood scent.

- (2) Base note: 3 drops sandalwood
- (0) Base note: 1 drop vanilla   *not commercial perfume*
- (0) Middle note: 8 drops grapefruit
- (2) Top note: 12 drops bergamot

Winter Wonderland Scent *Home Fragrance*

Here's a scent to put you in a wintery, holiday mood.

- Base note: 2 drops ginger
- Base note: 2 drops clove
- Middle note: 6 drops cinnamon
- Top note: 12 drops orange

Forest Scent *Home Fragrance*

Here's a wonderful woodsy, forest scent with a hint of peppermint.

- Base note: 20 drops cedarwood
- Middle note: 5 drops rosemary
- Middle note: 40 drops sweet orange
- Top note: 10 drops peppermint

Pumpkin Spice Scent *Home Scent*

- Base note: 1 drops clove
- Base note: 2 drops ginger
- Base note: 1 drop vanilla
- Middle note: 4 drops cinnamon
- Middle note: 4 drops nutmeg
- Top note: 12 drops orange

Woodland Wonder Scent *Home Scent*

This is another woodsy recipe.

- Base note: 4 drops cedarwood
- Middle note: 8 drops rosemary
- Top note: 6 drops orange
- Top note: 6 drops peppermint

Chai Scent *Home Scent*

This unusual scent has a fragrance that evokes chai.

- Base note: 4 drops clove
- Middle note: 4 drops cardamom

- Middle note: 4 drops cinnamon
- Top note: 12 drops sweet orange

Romantic Scent *Personal fragrance*

Here's a wonderfully classic romantic scent with a strong tone of rose.

- Base note: 4 drops vetiver
- Middle note: 8 drops rose
- Top note: 12 drops lime

may be missing the "not too familiar category"

Chapter 6 – Solid Perfume

Liquid perfumes aren't the only kind of organic perfume you can make at home. To make a solid perfume, you only need a few extra items and ingredients. In this chapter, we'll look at how to make a solid perfume, and provide recommendations on both recipes and supplies you need. Let's take a look!

Procedure

Here's what you need, in addition to 40 to 50 drops of your favorite essential oils:

- 2 tablespoons of beeswax
- 2 tablespoons of jojoba oil
- Small glass or metal jar (such as a lip balm tin, Altoid tin, lib balm tube, etc.)

Grate the beeswax and melt it over low heat and by putting a few inches of water in a saucepan, and then set a glass or ceramic container in the water – that will hold the beeswax while it melts.

Remove the beeswax from the heat, add jojoba oil to the melted beeswax and stir until thoroughly blended. Let the mixture cool to about 120°F, then add your essential oils. Be aware that this well set up quickly, so you want to have you oils blended and ready to add ahead of time. Once the blend has been mixed, store in a small glass jar and it's ready to use!

Note that you need to use equal parts beeswax and carrier oil. A typical lip balm container can hold about 2 tablespoons of beeswax and 2 tablespoons of carrier oil. As to the essential oils, you want to use 40 to 45 drops of oil to 2 tablespoons of beeswax and two tablespoons of carrier oil. You can use more oils to make the scent stronger, if you would like. The scent will mellow after you add it to the solid base.

Recipes

Here are some simple recipes for making solid perfumes. Note that the science behind combining the fragrances is the same for solid recipes as well as liquid perfume recipes.

Exciting

- Base note: 15 drops ginger
- Base note: 10 drops vetiver
- Middle note: 17 drops grapefruit

Sandalwood

- Base note: 12 drops sandalwood
- Base note: 12 drops vanilla

- Middle note: 15 drops grapefruit
- Top note: 12 drops bergamot

Sensuous

- Base note: 10 drops cedarwood
- Middle note: 15 drops ylang ylang
- Top note: 20 drops sweet orange

Intense

- Base note: 2 drops jasmine
- Middle note: 4 drops ylang-ylang
- Middle note: 3 drops rosewood
- Top note: 4 drops bergamot
- Top note: 6 drops orange

Garden

- Base note: 5 drops jasmine
- Middle note: 4 drops rose
- Middle note: 2 drops ylang ylang
- Top note: 2 drops cedar

Chapter 7 – Aromatherapy

When you use essential oils in your perfume, you can enjoy more than just a pleasant scent. This chapter discusses how you can use aromatherapy as part of your fragrance development, both in terms of fighting negative emotions and building positive atmospheres. We'll begin with what essential oils are recommended for achieving different effects, then provide a few sample recipes.

Essential Oils and Aromatherapy

Essential oils also can also have a positive, therapeutic effect on your emotions. The table below summarizes what essential oils are recommended for treating negative emotions.

Negative Emotion	Recommended Essential Oils
Depression	bergamot, lavender, geranium, grapefruit, jasmine, mandarin, neroli, lemon, rose, roman chamomile, ylang ylang, frankincense, orange, clary sage, sandalwood
Grief	rose, cypress, vetivier, frankincense, neroli, sandalwood
Loneliness	clary sage, chamomile (roman), rose, frankincense, bergamot
Fear	bergamot, clary sage, lemon, frankincense,

	grapefruit, jasmine, chamomile (roman), orange, sandalwood, vetiver, neroli, cedarwood
Insecurity	bergamot, sandalwood, cedarwood, vetiver, jasmine, frankincense
Panic Attacks	lavender, frankincense, neroli, rose
Weariness	patchouli, cypress, clary sage, sandalwood, frankincense, ginger, black pepper, jasmine, bergamot, lemon, grapefruit, peppermint, rosemary, vetiver, basil
Anger	vetiver, bergamot, rose, jasmine, , orange, patchouli, roman chamomile, ylang ylang, neroli

The following table summarizes essential oils recommended for achieving various positive emotions, such as creating an atmosphere of security or to support a peaceful, calm environment.

Positive Emotion	Recommended Essential Oils
Security	bergamot, jasmine, sandalwood, frankincense, vetiver, cedarwood
Pleasantness	lavender, sandalwood, neroli, roman chamomile, mandarin
Concentration	cypress, black pepper, lemon, peppermint, basil, rosemary
Peace	bergamot, lemon , neroli, orange, grapefruit, rose, sandalwood, ylang ylang, frankincense, geranium
Relaxation	clary sage, frankincense, bergamot, lavender, neroli, geranium, patchouli, roman chamomile,

| | sandalwood, vetiver, cedarwood, rose, mandarin |

Recipes

This can serve as a guide for choosing essential oils to achieve aromatherapy and fantastic, one-of-a-kind perfumes at the same time. With so many oils to choose from, you can easily create a pleasant scent to achieve positive emotions. Here is an example recipe to create a scent that has a peaceful, relaxing effect: sandalwood (base note), jasmine (middle note), and ylang ylang (middle note).

Here is possible combination for creating a joyous, happy atmosphere: clary sage (base note), chamomile (middle note), grapefruit (top note), sweet orange (top note), and lavender (top note).

Conclusion

If you've read up to this point, you're more than ready to start making your own customized organic perfumes that are economical, environmentally friendly, animal friendly, and fun! You know the benefits of organic perfumes, and you know why essential oils are a great way to begin.

You've got a good handle on the procedure, and you understand the importance of carrier oils to carry the scent and protect your skin, vodka to enable the essential oils to blend, and distilled water or spring water to dilute the final product. You also know it's important to allow your fragrances to cure to achieve the best effects.

You've learned the basic science behind developing fragrances, including fragrance notes, essential oil fragrance families, chypres, season scents, and more.

You also understand how the essential oils will evaporate at different rates from your skin, which means your fragrance will change as it remains on your skin. You also learned how to make solid perfumes, and have a good idea on what kinds of containers work the best for storing and using them.

You also learned about experimenting with scents, and what equipment is recommended for your own personal perfume laboratory.

You also had a crash course in aromatherapy, where you learned what essential oils are recommended for treating negative emotions such as anger or depression, as well as creating positive atmospheres of relaxing and energy.

You know what you need to have a great time making custom organic perfumes for yourself, your friends, and your family. We hope you have fun!

Made in the USA
Columbia, SC
24 September 2018